Mawe Albert DAKOUO

Quality of gentamycin injection in Bamako

Mawe Albert DAKOUO

Quality of gentamycin injection in Bamako

Evaluation of the quality of gentamycin injection dispensed in Bamako's health centers and pharmacies

ScienciaScripts

Imprint

Any brand names and product names mentioned in this book are subject to trademark, brand or patent protection and are trademarks or registered trademarks of their respective holders. The use of brand names, product names, common names, trade names, product descriptions etc. even without a particular marking in this work is in no way to be construed to mean that such names may be regarded as unrestricted in respect of trademark and brand protection legislation and could thus be used by anyone.

Cover image: www.ingimage.com

This book is a translation from the original published under ISBN 978-620-6-72056-0.

Publisher:
Sciencia Scripts
is a trademark of
Dodo Books Indian Ocean Ltd. and OmniScriptum S.R.L publishing group

120 High Road, East Finchley, London, N2 9ED, United Kingdom
Str. Armeneasca 28/1, office 1, Chisinau MD-2012, Republic of Moldova, Europe
Printed at: see last page
ISBN: 978-620-8-04111-3

DEDICACES

I dedicate this modest work

► To God

The Almighty, the Clement, the Merciful, who gave me life and granted me the chance to do this work. May I, Lord, serve you until the end of my life, and worship you and do only positive and constructive works.

ACKNOWLEDGEMENTS

► *To my father Fidèle DAKOUO*

Abi, Father, Patre, I love you in every language and every hour I've been near you I've grown up in peace and security, in joy and good humour. I owe my life to you, I owe my taste for happiness to you. You've been the best father and the best dad to me. My father, my most ardent wish is to keep you close to me for a long time to come. I want my children to have the chance to see a fabulous grandfather. A grandad who will give them everything he gave me. The wisdom, knowledge, generosity and respect you taught me. I remember that we spent days and nights learning from primary school right through to the baccalauréat, sometimes with a whip to back it up. I admit that it was very hard, but today, dear father, allow me to express my immense gratitude and my sincere thanks. Thank you, Father, thank you for everything, Dad! I'm immensely grateful to you, you're an exceptional person for me, my greatest opportunity.

► **To my mother Dabou Florence KONE**

Dear mother, I can't find the words to thank you today. This is the moment for me to thank Almighty God for giving us the chance to grow up with you. This work is the fruit of your patience, your sacrifices and your blessings.

► **To my brothers: Didi Vincent de Paul DAKOUO, Moussa DAKOUO, André DAKOUO**

► **To my sisters: Noellie DAKOUO, Reine Toumata DAKOUO, Clémentine Sohohan DAKOUO**

► *To my niece: Charlotte DAKOUO*

► *To my nephew: Kenikouo Barthélémy TOGO*

Brotherhood is priceless, as they say. I hope it will remain a sacred bond for us all. You have always been by my side, surrounding me with your affection, help and advice. I have never missed your love, encouragement and prayers. May God give us courage, long life and good health so that we can continue to share these moments of joy together. You have been exemplary to me in sharing all my worries and in sparing no effort to see me succeed. Words fail me to express all that I feel. Please accept the expression of my love and deep affection.

► **To the DAKOUO family of Madiakwy and KONE of Banconi and Ségou**

Because a child doesn't just belong to his or her biological parents, but to the whole family. Dad, mum, uncles, cousins, nieces and nephews, words can never express my gratitude enough. Over the years, you have given me unfailing support. You have always supported me in your prayers and encouraged me in my studies. Your presence, your advice and your generosity have filled my heart with love. I have not forgotten any of your kindnesses towards me. May God fill you with your blessings.

► *To the families: KOUMARE, COULIBALY,*

Your sympathy and support, both moral and material, have been invaluable to me in this work. Please accept my sincere gratitude.

► *To the late Drissa DIALLO*

Dear fellow students, thank you for the moments of joy and difficulty we have shared together; we have travelled the road of knowledge. Thank you for what we have been able to build together. I am proud to belong to this class.

► To my colleagues at the Nassouba pharmacy under the direction of Dr Abdoul Karim COULIBALY and Dr DOUYON Seydou, Dr Cheick Sidi Tahara DIAKITÉ, Dr Demba DIAKITÉ :

I thank God for giving me the chance to work with you.

► To my colleagues at Dr AG FAKIKE's Torokorobougou pharmacy, you will be engraved in my heart.

► To the staff of the LNS

Thank you from the bottom of my heart to everyone at the LNS, especially the Drug Quality Control Department. You welcomed me from the very first day of my internship. The whole process of analysing this study was made possible by your availability and collaboration. More than just a place to work, you provided me with the kind of support that a family should have. I am at a loss for words to express my deep gratitude, thank you to the great BENGALY, the great OUATTARA, uncle SAYON, aunt Marie Curie, DIAKITÉ Latifa, my brother Jacques DAKOUO, and my beloved aunt Niélé TRAORE. May God reward you.

TO OUR MASTER AND PRESIDENT OF THE JURY

Professor Sékou BAH

► *Full Professor of Pharmacology at the FMOS /FAPH ;*

► *Member of the Technical Pharmacovigilance Committee ;*

► *Master's degree in international community health;*

► *Head of the Hospital Pharmacy Department at the Point G University Hospital;*

► *Vice Dean of the Faculty of Pharmacy (FAPH)*

Honourable Master,

It is a great honour and an immense pleasure for us that you have agreed to chair this jury, despite your many requests. Your simplicity, your wisdom, your availability and your ability to listen and analyse, your concern for a job well done and your scientific rigour are professional qualities that have aroused our admiration and confidence. Please accept, dear Master, the expression of our deepest gratitude.

TO OUR TEACHER AND JURY MEMBER

Dr Dominique Patomo ARAMA

► *Lecturer at the Faculty of Pharmacy, USTTB;*

► *Executive Vice President, Pharmaceuticals and Medicines ;*

► *Member of the WAHO Expert Committee on Product Certification pharmaceuticals ;*

► *Certified in practical knowledge and management of medical devices ;*

► *Silver Star of National Merit with Lion Standing Effigy.*

Dear Master,

We would like to thank you very much for your willingness and friendliness in judging our work. Your scientific and human qualities make you a modest and exemplary supervisor. In the hope that this work will meet your expectations, please be assured, dear Master, of our complete availability and receive the expression of our deepest gratitude.

TO OUR MASTER AND SUPERVISOR

Professor Benoît Yaranga KOUMARE

► *Pharmacist, Professor of Analytical Chemistry/Bromatology at the USTTB;*

► *Director General of the National Health Laboratory in Bamako ;*

► *Specialist in Quality Assurance and Quality Control of Medicines / Pharmacotherapy (rational prescription of medicines) and neuropharmacology;*

► *Expert analyst and pharmacologist with the Commission Nationale*

d'Autorisation de Mise sur le Marché des Médicaments au Mali (CNAMM);

► *Quality expert for the Regional Veterinary Medicines Committee within the*

UEMOA ;

► *Member of the Société Ouest Africaine de Chimie (SOACHIM);*

► *Medal-holder, Knight of the Order of Merit for Health in Mali.*

Dear Master,

I am infinitely grateful to you for your investment in this work and for the confidence you have shown in allowing me to work on this thesis. Your friendliness, seriousness, competence, pragmatism and, above all, your human qualities have left a lasting impression on me. We are proud to have benefited from your training. We will always remember you as an excellent teacher and a professional worthy of respect.

TABLE OF CONTENTS

INTRODUCTION

The medicines market has changed considerably in recent years. Free movement of medicines has given rise to a number of difficulties, including the loss of control over the quality of certain products. It is against this backdrop that the concepts of counterfeit and misbranded medicines and the irrational use of medicines have emerged. It should also be emphasised that these two scourges, linked to the constant increase in the illegal trade in medicines, are the main causes of therapeutic inefficiency (1).

The presence of substandard or falsified medical products in countries and their use by patients threatens to undermine progress towards achieving sustainable development goals. These products may be of insufficient quality, unsafe or ineffective, threatening the health of those who take them. The problem of substandard or falsified medical products continues to grow with the increasing complexity of globalised manufacturing and distribution systems. This complexity increases the risk of production errors or of medicines deteriorating between the factory and the consumer. The growth in demand for medicines, vaccines and other medical products in almost all countries, combined with poorly managed supply chains and increased trade, provides opportunities for falsified medicines to enter supply chains (2).

In low- and middle-income countries, an estimated 10% of medical products are substandard or falsified. Based on the WHO model using these data, up to 72,430 deaths from childhood pneumonia can be attributed to the use of substandard/falsified medicines (2). The 2019 World Health Assembly report estimates that barely 30% of national regulatory authorities worldwide have the capacity to perform all essential regulatory functions for medicines (3).

Another study on the Creation of the African Medicines Agency (AMA): progress, challenges and regulatory preparedness estimates that only 7% of African countries have moderately developed regulatory capacity, and over 90% have little or no capacity (4).

Gentamicin is produced by micro-organisms of the Micromonospora genus, the main producer being the actinomycete bacterium Micromonospora echinospora (5).

Gentamicin was first approved by the Food and Drug Administration for intramuscular (IM) use in 1969 and intravenous (IV) use in 1971 (5). It is generally used as a curative treatment in combination with beta-lactam antibiotics. However, it can also be prescribed as monotherapy in certain clinical situations, particularly for the treatment of Gram-negative bacterial infections. In these cases, it is an important weapon for the therapeutic clinician because of its efficacy in the treatment of urinary tract infections.

Today, however, the effectiveness of antibiotics is seriously affected by the emergence of antimicrobial resistance. As defined by the World Health Organisation (WHO), resistance "occurs when bacteria, viruses, fungi and parasites evolve over time and no longer respond to drugs, making the treatment of infections more complex and increasing the risk of spread, severe disease and death". Similarly, antibiotic resistance occurs when bacteria evolve in response to inappropriate use of antibiotics, with inhibitory pressure becoming insufficient (6). Resistant bacteria, found in hospitals but also in the community, therefore lead to an increase in morbidity and mortality. This phenomenon is now considered to be one of the biggest public health problems in the world (6). Mali has to face up to the emergence of this problem. Murray and colleagues have shown that the West African region has the highest death rate associated with antimicrobial resistance (more than 100 deaths per 100,000) (6). In a world marked by an increase in chemoresistance, leading to the adoption of combination therapies, the advent of multi-source generic medicines, and the spread of counterfeit and poor-quality medicines, often without active ingredients or with falsified active ingredients, the pharmaceutical regulatory authorities need to be more vigilant. Guaranteeing the quality of pharmaceutical products, whether manufactured locally or imported, is fundamental to any healthcare system. The use of ineffective, poor-quality and harmful medicines can lead to therapeutic failure, disease exacerbation, drug resistance and even death. It also contributes to reducing consumer confidence in healthcare systems, healthcare providers, manufacturers and distributors of pharmaceutical products (2).

Strategic objective 4 of the NAP aims to optimise the use of antimicrobial agents in healthcare

human, animal, environmental and plant production(7).

For a drug-importing country like Mali, it is essential to ensure that the injectable gentamicin dispensed in Mali's health centres and private pharmacies is of good quality. It was with this in mind that we undertook this study, which looked at the quality of o f injectable gentamicin dispensed in health centres and private pharmacies in the District of Bamako.

OBJECTIVES

1. OBJECTIVE

To assess the quality of injectable gentamicin dispensed in health centres and private pharmacies in Bamako.

2. SPECIFIC OBJECTIVES

√ Determine the prevalence of low-grade gentamicin in circulation in selected healthcare institutions;

√ Determine the recording status of the sampled gentamicin;

√ Provide quality gentamicin data to the DPM for possible regulatory/administrative action.

GENERAL

3. National Pharmaceutical Policy

Mali has a National Pharmaceutical Policy (NPP) adopted in 1999. It was revised in 2012. The general objective of this policy is to guarantee equitable access to quality essential medicines for the population and to promote their rational use.

In order to ensure an adequate supply of healthcare products for the population, a Master Plan for the Supply of Essential Medicines (SDAME) was drawn up in 1995 and revised in 2010 to become the Master Plan for the Supply and Distribution of Essential Medicines (SDADME). It describes the supply system and the roles and responsibilities of players at different levels of the health pyramid. Decision No. 2011-774/MS-SG of 11 July 2011 makes application of the SDADME mandatory. The aim of the SDADME is to ensure the correct supply of health products to the population throughout the national territory.

In Mali, healthcare products are supplied by the Pharmacie Populaire du Mali (PPM), which is the State's preferred tool for the supply, storage and distribution of healthcare products under a State-PPM contract plan. This system is supplemented by the private sector through pharmaceutical product import and wholesale establishments, also known as private wholesalers (8).

4. Master plan for the supply and distribution of essential medicines

-Health Products (SDADME-PS)

Mechanism that describes the practical and functional measures that should enable health facilities to ensure a correct and continuous supply of essential medicines and other quality health products that are accessible to communities (8).

4.1. SDADME Implementation Principles- PS

- Cost recovery and community involvement in the management of health products;

- Controlling needs at each level: the various levels (PPM, Hospitals, CSRéf, CSCom) are each responsible for continuously estimating their needs in terms of healthcare products, services and equipment.

orders, purchasing and management ;

- Determining and setting up initial stocks: constituting working capital ;

- Strengthening the distribution network, to bring healthcare products closer to users and reduce approach costs and the risk of stock-outs, a network has been defined as follows: central shops (PPM); regional shops (PPM), pharmacies, etc.hospitals, DRCs, DVs and private establishments importing and wholesaling products pharmaceuticals ;

- To optimise distribution, supply is based on the most suitable structure. more accessible: Magasin Régional de la Pharmacie Populaire du Mali (MR-PPM), Dépôt Répartiteur de Cercle (DRC).

- National procurement procedures (calls for tender, etc.) following an annual procurement plan: to guarantee the affordability and quality of healthcare products.

• The integration within the SDADME-PS of the management of all healthcare products, whether paid for by patients or free of charge, in order to control consumption requirements and guarantee their availability and quality through the application of best practices. professional.

• Strengthening the management of the entire system: definition of a chart of accounts, community involvement ;

• The quality control and inspection organisation;

• Greater availability of essential generic INN medicines in the private sector;

• Training and information for stakeholders ;

• Information and education for beneficiaries: this should cover essential medicines in INN form, their properties, their benefits, precautions for use, the services that provide them and the benefits of cost recovery;

• Active" monitoring and reinforcement through operational research: through ongoing evaluation using relevant indicators, and the organisation of operational research on themes that will help to clarify certain issues and help to readjust the strategies(8).

5. Medicines

A medicinal product is defined as any substance or composition presented as having curative or preventive properties in respect of human or animal diseases, as well as any product which may be administered to human beings or animals with a view to making a medical diagnosis or to restoring, correcting or modifying their organic function (8).

5.1. Components of a medicine

Medicines are made up of three main components:

5.1.1. Active principle

It is a substance of chemical or natural origin with a specific curative or preventive mechanism of action. In other words, it is the element that possesses the curative or preventive pharmacological properties of the drug. It is always the active principle that is called the medicine. These substances are intended to have a pharmacological action or any other direct effect for the diagnosis, cure, mitigation, treatment or prevention of a disease, or to affect the structure and function of the body.

5.1.2. Excipient

An excipient is a substance or mixture of substances of chemical or natural origin, inactive in themselves against disease, which, when used in the formulation, facilitates the preparation and use of the medicinal product. The excipient may also play an important role in the release of the active ingredient from the medicinal product, thereby modifying its therapeutic activity. Examples of excipients include modified starches and modified celluloses, which are disintegrating agents used in dry forms (tablets, capsules, etc.) to accelerate their disintegration (or disintegration) once they reach the stomach.

5.1.3. Packaging

All the material elements designed to protect the medicinal product throughout its life; a distinction is made between the primary packaging in contact with the medicinal product and the secondary packaging which is not in contact with the medicinal product and which complements the primary packaging (9).

5.2. Names of medicines

According to the WHO, this is the globally recognised name for each pharmaceutical substance, replacing its rarely simple chemical name. A medicine has a chemical name, an international non-proprietary name (INN) and a trade name (10,11).

5.2.1. Chemical name

The chemical or scientific name corresponds to the chemical formula of the substance that makes up the medicine.

5.2.2. International Non-proprietary Name (INN)

The International Non-proprietary Name (INN) or generic name is assigned by the WHO. This name is made up of key segments that provide information on the origin and pharmacological mode of action of the product.

5.2.3. Trade name

The brand or pharmaceutical name is chosen by the manufacturer of the medicine. This name is generally short and easy to remember, but unlike the INN, it may differ from one country to another for the same medicine.

5.3. Different forms of medicines

The "form" of a medicine does not refer solely to its physical appearance. It refers to all the parameters given to it during manufacture. The term "form" is an abbreviation of the expression "galenic form", referring to galenic pharmacy, which is the "science and art of preparing, preserving and presenting medicines". It is named after the Greek physician Galen (12). Existing forms are generally classified according to the **route of administration of** the drug.

5.3.1. Oral forms of medicines ;

Swallowable medicines take the form of :

• Liquid, such as syrups, solutions (or drops, often diluted in a glass of water), etc. ;

• Solid, such as tablets, pills, pastilles, capsules, granules, powders, etc.

5.3.2. Dermal or transdermal forms

These drugs are administered by **the skin**: they are applied to the skin in the same way as creams, ointments, gels, etc. The patch, which is stuck to the skin, is a transdermal device that allows the drug to pass slowly and evenly through the skin before entering the bloodstream.

5.3.3. Injectable forms of medicines

Medicines administered **by injection** take the form of solid implants or liquids for injections :

• Intravenous ;

• Intramuscular ;

• Or subcutaneous.

5.3.4. Drug forms that pass through mucous membranes

There are several routes for administering drugs through the mucous membranes:

• The **perlingual route**, which involves allowing the medicine to melt under the tongue, such as certain tablets or solutions (particularly in powder form);
• The **nasal route**. These medicines are put into the nose: solutions, powders, ointments, creams;
• The **pulmonary route**, such as inhalation ;

• **Rectal route** such as suppositories, certain liquids or specific foams;

• The **vaginal route:** this refers to ova, tablets or capsules that pass through the vaginal mucosa;
• **Ocular route**: eye drops, ointments, creams, washing solutions, artificial tears, etc., to be applied to the eyes.
• The **auricular route**. These medicines are placed in the ear canal: ear drops, ointments, creams (12).

5.4. Categories of medicines

Depending on the origin of their preparation formulas, we have :

► Magistral medicinal product: This is any preparation made by a pharmacist in his dispensary on the basis of a formula detailed in a medical prescription (13).
► Compendial medicinal product: This is a preparation whose composition and method of preparation are listed in the pharmacopoeia or in a national formulary (13).
► Speciality medicine: This is a medicine prepared in advance, presented in a specific pack, marketed under a special name and intended to be dispensed in several pharmacies (13).
► Generic medicinal product: Generic medicinal product refers to any proprietary medicinal product whose patent has expired and entered the public domain (8).
► Improved traditional medicines: These are medicines derived from the local traditional pharmacopoeia, with defined toxicity limits, pharmacological activity confirmed by scientific research, quantified dosage and controlled quality when they are placed on the market (8).

5.5. Lot and number of lot

► **Batch:** the batch is the quantity of a medicinal product manufactured during a given production cycle. or production. The essential quality of a production batch is its homogeneity.

► **Batch number:** the batch number is the designation (printed on the label of a medicinal product in the form of numbers and/or letters) which makes it possible to identify the batch to which a specific box of medicinal product belongs, and it is from this number that production and distribution traceability can be established. For various reasons, a laboratory may

be obliged to recall medicines, and it is thanks to this batch number that the batch recall can be performed (9).

5.6. Essential medicines

An essential drug is any product whose efficacy and safety have been scientifically demonstrated, and which is essential for providing basic preventive and curative healthcare for around 80% of local pathologies (8).

6. Notion of infringement

6.1. Definition :

According to the WHO, "A counterfeit medicine is one that is deliberately and fraudulently mislabelled to indicate its identity and/or true source". It may be a speciality or a generic product, and among counterfeit products there are those that contain the right ingredients and others that contain the wrong ingredients, or even no active ingredient at all. Others contain insufficient active ingredient and their packaging has been tampered with (14).

Counterfeiting may involve a reference product (brand name) or a generic medicine. It can take a variety of forms: identical presentation and/or composition; different composition (absence, under- or overdosage of active ingredient, presence of harmful ingredients); falsified packaging (counterfeit packaging, for example to "push back" the expiry date of expired medicines).

6.2. Falsified

The World Health Organisation (WHO) defines a falsified medicine as one whose identity, composition or source are deliberately and fraudulently misrepresented. Unknown manufacturers produce these medicines in unsanitary and uncontrolled conditions. They may contain harmful contaminants, inactive components (such as chalk or corn or potato starch), the wrong API or the wrong amount of the correct API, or no API at all. Falsified medicines often have virtually the same packaging as the genuine medicine, making it difficult to distinguish between the two without carrying out detection tests on the ingredients of the medicine.

(15). A falsified medicinal product is any medicinal product with a false presentation of at least one of the following characteristics:

■ Its identity, including its packaging and labelling, its name or composition in the case of any of its constituents, including excipients, and the dosage of these constituents;

■ Its source, including its manufacturer, country of manufacture, country of origin or

the marketing authorisation holder ;

■ Its history, including records and documents relating to the distribution channels used (16).

6.3.Medicines of inferior quality

The WHO defines a substandard medicine, also known as "off-spec", as an authorised medical product that does not meet its quality standards or specifications, or both. They are essentially manufactured by reputable manufacturers with no intention of deceiving or ripping off the patient (15).

7. AMINOGLYCOSIDES

7.1. Introduction

Aminoglycosides or aminosides are amino sugars which, depending on their chemical structure, can be divided into two main groups: streptomycin and its derivatives on the one hand, and the 2-deoxystreptamine group on the other. These are basic, water-soluble organic compounds with a molecular weight of 500 to 800 DA. Their optimal antibacterial activity occurs at a pH of 7.5 to 8.5. Aminoglycosides are rapidly bactericidal antibiotics, acting in particular on aerobic Gram-negative bacilli, staphylococci and Gram-positive bacilli. They are weakly active or inactive against anaerobes, streptococci and pneumococci. Their combination with B-lactam antibiotics, fluoroquinolones and polypeptide antibiotics is synergistic (17).

7.2. Classification

Aminoglycosides can be divided into two groups (Table 1).

■ Streptomycin and its derivatives, combining streptidine with a pentose and a glucosamine

■ Deoxystreptamines, divided into two groups depending on whether the substitutions occur in the 4,5 or 4,6 position.

Table I: Distribution of aminoglycosides

Deoxystreptamines		Other
4,5-Bisubstituted4	,6-Bisubstituted	
	NeomycinKanamycins A, B, C	Streptomycin
Ribostamycin	Dideoxykanamycin	Spectinomycin
Lividomycin	Tobramycin	Apramycin
Paromomycin	**Gentamicin**	Fortimicin
ButiromycinSisomicin Isepamicin	, Netilmicin, Amikacin, Sagamicin, Dibekacin, Arbecacin	

7.3. Mechanism of action

Kasugamicin Istamicin Dactomycin They essentially act on the bacterial ribosome by interfering with the reading of the genetic code and inhibiting all stages of protein synthesis. They are bactericidal.Their bactericidal activity is generally concentration-dependent, and there is a post-antibiotic effect. These two properties, combined with a reduction in toxicity, explain the reduction in the number of injections for the same daily dosage.
The majority of studies into their mode of action have been undertaken with streptomycin. The ribosome has been identified as the preferred target of all the aminoglycosides tested. Ribosome alterations were observed in the mutants, and the ribosomal proteins affected by the mutation were identified and characterised. Although the ribosome has been identified as the main target of aminoglycoside action, studies into the exact mode of action are complicated by the fact that these products (kanamycin and gentamicin have the same action as streptomycin)

have different and apparently unrelated effects on bacteria in culture. For example, membrane modifications, inhibition of protein synthesis, modifications to RNA synthesis and morphological changes have been observed.

Inhibition of protein synthesis at the ribosomal level is the most likely mechanism of action of aminoglycosides. Concomitant effects contribute to bactericidal activity, as aminoglycosides concentrated in the cell are capable of producing lethal effects, due in particular to the role of membrane modifications.

7.4.Structure-activity relationships of aminoglycosides

A number of studies have been carried out on the structure-activity relationship of aminoglycosides. Initial studies with streptomycin suggest that the number of amino groups determines the efficacy of the compound. However, other groups are just as important.

In this way, streptamine replaces deoxystreptamine without affecting the efficacy of neomycin. Fortimicin contains neither streptamine nor deoxystreptamine, but its structure contains groups whose arrangement results in identical behaviour towards ribosomal receptors. Compounds containing an epistreptamine group are less active, but other modifications of the deoxystreptamine ring do not necessarily alter the activity of the product. This cycle is very important, but it is not the only factor in activity (15).

Other structural modifications are known. The loss of a hydroxyl group does not alter activity against the ribosome but does affect the antibacterial spectrum of the aminoglycoside. The superior activity of gentamicin and tobramycin against Pseudomonas aeruginosa appears to be linked to differences in the transport properties of 3'-OH and 3'-deoxy compounds. The antipseudomonas activity of amikacin is enhanced by protection against enzymatic inactivation by substitution on the amino group.

Other structural modifications can lead to changes in the spectrum of aminoglycosides. For example, against resistant strains, structural changes can restrict the activity of inactivating enzymes. The number of amino groups affects the activity of compounds, and some are more important than others. This is the case with 6', which is more important than 2'. Thus, kanamycin B with a 2',6-diamino sugar is more active than kanamycin A with a 2'-amino sugar.

7.5.Resistance mechanisms

Some bacteria may be naturally and consistently resistant to aminoglycosides, in particular obligate anaerobes such as Bacteroides and Clostridium, or certain aerobes and anaerobes such as Streptococcus pyogenes, Streptococcus pneumoniae and Enterococcus faecalis. For streptococci as a whole, resistance is low, between 16 and 256 mg/litre for streptomycin and between 4 and 128 mg/litre for gentamicin, and this low level can be explained by inefficient active transport across the bacterial membrane. Treponema, Leptospira and Actinomycetes spp. are naturally resistant to aminoglycosides. Bacteria can acquire resistance to aminoglycosides, and this phenomenon was exacerbated in the years between 1985 and 1990. Resistance can be acquired through four mechanisms:

■ alteration of the target,

■ interference with antibiotic transport (efflux),

■ enzymatic inhibition of the antibiotic, and

■ target substitution.

The first three mechanisms are secondary to chromosomal or plasmid-mediated mutations. The fourth is only observed after the acquisition of plasmid or transposon resistance. Resistance to aminoglycosides can occur after a mutation (alteration-interference) or after the acquisition of a plasmid (enzymatic action). Alteration of the ribosomal target is linked to a mutation, with the substitution of a single amino acid causing a reduction in the affinity of the ribosome for the aminoglycoside. This often leads to strong resistance from the outset. This resistance is not cross-linked between aminoglycosides, given the multiplicity of binding sites. The modifications encountered are acetylation, phosphorylation and adenylation. (Note: adenylic acid = adenosine 5-phosphate; adelylation involves binding via the phosphate). The enzymes are called AAC (aminoglycoside acetyltransferase), APH (aminoside phosphotransferase) and ANT (aminoside nucleotidyltransferase) (sometimes AAD, aminoside adenylyltransferase). They differ in the reaction they catalyse, the derivatisation position (Figure 1).

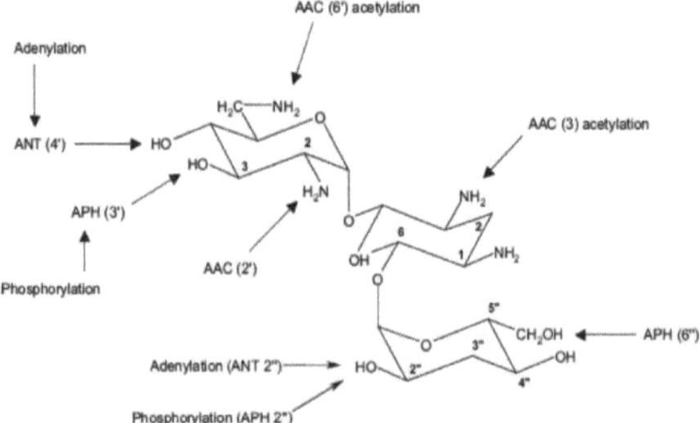

Figure 1: Sites of enzymatic inactivation of aminoglycosides

7.6. Pharmacology

⤹ Absorption

Absorption is complete after intramuscular administration. There is little or no protein binding. The apparent elimination half-life is approximately 2 hours and elimination is predominantly renal, with glomerular filtration and tubular reabsorption. Elimination pharmacokinetics are independent of dose and route of administration. Tissue diffusion is low, but renal accumulation occurs, particularly in the cortex. Renal insufficiency causes a marked increase in elimination half-life and requires dosage adjustment. Gentamicin, tobramycin, sisomicin, netilmicin and dibekacin are administered clinically at a unit dose of 1 to 2 mg/kg body weight. Maximum serum concentrations obtained after intramuscular injection are between 4 and 7 mg/litre.

Streptomycin, kanamycin and amikacin are prescribed clinically in unit doses of around 7.5 mg/kg (500 mg). Maximum serum concentrations are between 15 and 25 mg/litre. The serum distribution half-life is between 0.20 and 0.40 hours for all aminoglycosides. Pharmacokinetic studies in the same subjects at different doses have shown that pharmacokinetics are independent of dose. Concentration and area under the curves are proportional to dose and are not affected by dosing regimen or elimination half-life. This, combined with efficacy and toxicity studies, is an argument in favour of once-daily administration.

Metabolism and excretion

Biotransformation of aminoglycosides is negligible (10%). They are found almost entirely in unchanged and biologically active form in the urine.

Biliary excretion

The biliary route is only a very secondary route of elimination for aminoglycosides (0.5 to 2

% of the dose administered dose) without enterohepatic cycling. For this reason, hepatobiliary disorders have little effect on elimination. Effective biliary concentrations of kanamycin, gentamicin and tobramycin have been found in patients without biliary obstruction. Conversely, penetration of the bile ducts is poor in the presence of gallstones or severe hepatic insufficiency.

Renal elimination

The renal route is the main route of elimination for aminoglycosides. Urinary concentrations are very high and elimination is rapid. Eighty to 90% of the dose administered is recovered in the urine within 24 hours. The administration of a probenecid does not affect elimination, which tends to prove the absence of tubular secretion. Aminoglycosides are eliminated by glomerular filtration and are partly reabsorbed in the proximal tubule. For this reason, renal clearance is lower than creatinine clearance (CLCR). Total serum clearance is similar to renal clearance, confirming the absence of metabolism.

7.7. Gentamicin

Gentamicin is an aminoglycoside antibiotic. It is a bactericidal inhibitor of protein synthesis. Its main use is to treat infections caused by aerobic Gram-negative bacteria. The active ingredient is a complex of oligosaccharides, the core of which is deoxystreptamine, obtained by fermentation of single-spored actinomycetes of the genus Micromonospora. Gentamicin is a mixture of three components with approximately the same activity (Figure 2).

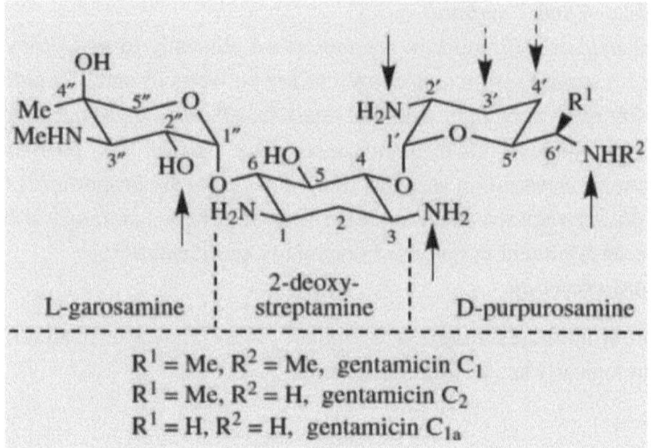

Figure 2: General structure of gentamicin The natural antibacterial spectrum of gentamicin is as follows:

- The species usually susceptible are gram-negative bacilli, gram-positive bacilli and meticillin-sensitive staphylococci;
- the species that are usually resistant are streptococci, pneumonococci, fungi and viruses.

meningococci, tubercle bacilli, treponemes and anaerobic germs.

When gentamicin is administered orally at therapeutic doses, it virtually does not cross the digestive barrier. When administered parenterally, gentamicin diffuses into all tissues except the prostate. It does not cross the blood-brain barrier. It is administered by the intramuscular or intravenous route as a discontinuous infusion over a period of 30 to 60 minutes.Binding to plasma proteins is low (0 to 3%). Elimination is rapid, in 6 to 8 hours, by glomerular filtration in the unchanged and therefore active form. The half-life is 2 to 4 hours in normorenal adults and 3 to 6 hours in infants and neonates. Gentamicin sulphate solution is a sterile injectable solution generally supplied in vials or ampoules. Gentamicin is a fermentation product supplied as a sulphate salt. This salt is manufactured into a sterile injectable solution using a standard formulation and filling/finishing process. The critical aspect of this manufacture is to maintain the sterility of the product.Gentamicin Injection is a sterile solution of gentamicin sulphate in water for injection and is mainly available in 2 mL vials or ampoules in two strengths (10 mg/mL or 40 mg/mL) for parenteral administration. Gentamicin sulphate, a water-soluble antibiotic of the aminoglycoside group, is a sulphate salt of the gentamicin fractions C1, C1a C2 and C2a, derived from the growth of Micromonospora echinospora, an actinomycete. It is a clear, colourless and odourless solution diluted in 0.9% sodium chloride or 5% glucose solution. It was patented in 1962 and approved for medical use in 1964. Gentamicin is one of the most frequently prescribed aminoglycosides, due to its broad spectrum of action, low cost and high availability. It is effective against both Gram-positive and Gram-negative organisms, but is particularly useful for treating Gram-negative infections (18).The main toxicities of gentamicin are ototoxicity and nephrotoxicity. Unfortunately, gentamicin ototoxicity is in many cases irreversible. Nephrotoxicity is generally reversible.

Precautions for safe handling include avoiding contact with concentrated solutions (19).

8. AWaRe classification :

+ Challenge to the AWaRe classification of antibiotics

√ Worldwide, the use of antimicrobials is suffering from :

• Overuse due to poor prescribing practices (in many contexts, more

50% of antibiotic prescriptions are inappropriate)

• Under-utilisation due to lack of access to the necessary drugs.

√ Factors contributing to the sub-optimal use of ATBs include :

• Lack of knowledge and awareness among prescribers and the public

• Limited access to diagnostic tests and insufficient diagnostic capacity

• Lack of access to data-based treatment guidelines

• Lack of access to data on the quality of prescribing and use of ATBs

• Preference for the use of broad-spectrum antibiotics, even if alternative broad-spectrum antibiotics are available.

are available(20)

+ AWaRe classification developed by the WHO

The AWaRe classification developed by the WHO follows a series of recommendations, facilitating the classification of ATBs with a view to their inclusion in the national list of essential medicines.
This approach categorises the different antibiotics into 3 classes:

√ Access to antibiotics group (A)

√ Antibiotics Watch Group (Wa)

√ Reserve" group of antibiotics (Re) Not included in the AWaRe TBA :
√ Anti-leprosy drugs

√ Anti-tuberculosis drugs

• **ACCESS**

These are the antibiotics of choice for the 25 most common infectious diseases. They are affordable, of controlled quality and must be available at all times.
They are :

√ First-line antibiotics (sensitive narrow-spectrum TBAs with low toxicity and the potential to develop resistance);
√ Second-line antibiotics (sensitive TBAs with a broader spectrum, increased risk of toxicity or development of resistance)

Lower priority for activities to promote correct use Example: Amoxicillin, **Gentamicin**, Amikacin, Metronidazole etc.

- **WATCH (SURVEILLANCE)**

These are "high-priority and critically important antimicrobials" for human health. and animal, they are recommended only for specific and limited indications (20).

It includes susceptible TBAs with potentially higher toxicity or greater potential for the development of resistance, which must not be used for prophylactic purposes in animals or in agricultural production. They should be the target of activities to promote proper use, and their use should be actively monitored by occasional prevalence surveys(20).
For example: Azithromycin, Ciprofloxacin, Ceftriaxone, Cefixime, etc.

- **RESERVE**

They should be used as a last resort, when all other antibiotics have failed or cannot be used because of contraindications, and should be available when needed(20). Their use is strictly limited to very specific patients and clinical contexts. These are the new generations of ATBs and are protected and targeted as a priority by activities to promote correct use, centralised monitoring and reporting (20).
Example: Ceftazidime + Azibactam, Meropeneme + Vaborbactam, Polymycin B, Fosfomycin (IV) etc.

9. CONCEPTS OF QUALITY ASSURANCE

Quality assurance is defined as an integrated system of activities involving planning, quality control, quality assessment, quality reporting and quality improvement to ensure that a product or service meets defined quality standards with a stated level of confidence (21).
Quality assurance in the pharmaceutical industry takes place upstream and downstream, at every stage of production, from the control of raw materials (active ingredients and excipients), the application of good manufacturing practice (GMP) in all operations through to control of the finished product in the laboratory, not forgetting the attention paid to packaging(22).

9.1. Quality standards

Specifications are a set of carefully selected standards and analytical methods that can be used to assess the integrity of medicinal products or dosage forms and raw materials. To ensure the uniformity of all batches of a medicinal product in one or more dosage forms, it is necessary to establish appropriate standards for identity, purity, strength, behaviour and other characteristics. Strict adherence to these standards is the key to achieving the desired quality (21).

9.2. Control Quality

All measures taken, including specification, sampling, testing and analytical authorisation, to ensure that raw materials, intermediates, packaging materials and finished pharmaceutical products comply with established specifications for identity, assay, purity and other characteristics. This includes:

• The inspection of product manufacturing facilities and the inspection of

quality control to ensure that medicines are manufactured in accordance with GMP rules;

• Control of raw materials and excipients ;

• Checking the integrity of medicines before and after distribution;

• Control of imported medicines at the point of entry and thereafter.

All these activities are based on the collection and quality assessment of samples of medicinal products, to check that they meet the quality standards established to determine their acceptability(21).

9.3. Post-marketing surveillance

Surveillance activities that take place following market approval of a medicinal product, including: maintenance of product authorisation and/or registration of variations or renewals; regular inspections of manufacturers, wholesalers, distributors and retailers; quality control testing; pharmacovigilance; control of promotion; public reporting of poor quality products; handling of market complaints; removal and disposal of non-compliant products. Post-marketing surveillance (PMS) is generally regarded as a key regulatory function and refers to the full range of quality surveillance activities.

9.4. Good Manufacturing Practices (GMP) for medicines

Part of quality assurance which ensures that medicinal products are always produced and controlled in compliance with the quality standards appropriate to their intended purpose and in accordance with the conditions of the marketing authorisation (23).Before any medicine is put on sale, it is produced by a manufacturing laboratory that must comply with GMP. These are the elements of quality assurance recommended by the WHO (24). GMP ensures that products are manufactured and controlled in a uniform manner and to the quality standards appropriate to their use and specified in the marketing authorisation. GMPs cover all aspects of production and encompass the material used, the premises and staff hygiene. These practices help to minimise risks in the pharmaceutical manufacturing process.

9.5.WHO certification system (Prequalification)

WHO Prequalification aims to ensure access to key health products that meet global standards of quality, safety and efficacy/performance, in order to optimise the use of health resources and improve health outcomes.

These are activities undertaken to define the need for a product or service, to solicit expressions of interest from companies wishing to provide the service or product in question, and to examine the product or service offered against technical specifications, and the facility where the product or service is prepared, with reference to current Good Manufacturing Practice (GMP) standards. Prequalification is required for all medicinal products, whatever their composition and wherever they are manufactured/licensed.

(25). WHO prequalification of laboratories has become a reliable and reputable symbol of safety, quality and efficiency among stakeholders.

9.6.System ISO

ISO (International Organization for Standardization) is an independent, non-governmental organization consisting of 162 national standards bodies. Through its members, the Organization brings together experts who pool their knowledge to develop voluntary International Standards that are consensus-based, market-relevant, support innovation and provide solutions to global challenges. To date, ISO has published more than 21 500 International Standards and related publications, covering almost every sector, from technology to food safety, agriculture and health.

ISO/IEC 17025 is an international reference for testing and calibration laboratories wishing to demonstrate their ability to produce reliable results.

• It enables laboratories to demonstrate that they are operating competently and producing valid results, thereby boosting confidence in their work, both nationally and globally.

• It also contributes to facilitating cooperation between laboratories and other organisations, in particular by facilitating wider acceptance of results between countries.

• It also allows test reports and certificates to be accepted from one country to another without the need for further testing, a measure that facilitates international trade. WHO pre-qualification and the ISO system enable organisations to have the necessary next certificates

Registration : A procedure by which a registration body indicates the relevant characteristics of a product, process or service, or details of an organisation or person, on an appropriate publicly available list or a procedure used to give written assurance that a system conforms to specified requirements.

Accreditation: procedure by which an authoritative body formally recognizes that an organization or person is competent to carry out specific tasks **Certification:** procedure for providing written assurance that a product, process, service or person's qualifications conform to specified requirements.

9.7. Marketing authorisation Market

As its name suggests, this is an authorisation issued by the competent authority of a country for the sale of a product on the national market after assessment of its safety, efficacy and quality. Any medicine sold in a country must obtain marketing authorisation. In order to obtain this authorisation, the MA applicant must prepare a dossier in which he must provide :

• The safety of the product for humans ;

• Product effectiveness;

• Side effects and toxicity.

The marketing authorisation provides information that makes it possible to control the quality, efficacy and safety of a product. It provides information on the raw materials used, the composition and detailed formulation of the product, identification of its active ingredients, chemical interchangeability, packaging, shelf life and labelling (26).

10. General method for analysing medicines

The quality o f a medicinal product is assessed in the laboratory on both the packaging and the product it contains. The stages of an inspection are as follows:

► Traceability: in each control laboratory, a search is first carried out in the database to find out whether the product has indeed been manufactured by a site of the company that appears on the packaging. Analyses are carried out on the batch number, date of manufacture, etc.

► Visual examination of the packaging: this involves analysis of the printing fonts, engraving impressions, glue tabs on the boxes, etc. All these elements are compared by imaging with the real reference.

► General chemical analysis: during this analysis, spectroscopic techniques are used to determine the composition of the product and compare it with the characteristics of references recorded in a database.

► Precise chemical analysis: this is the last stage if the counterfeit is proven. It enables a more detailed chemical analysis to be carried out and to determine whether the active ingredient, toxic products, etc. are present in the product. The techniques used here are most often liquid or gas chromatography techniques, which enable unknown compounds to be identified in large quantities or in trace amounts.

8.1. Analysis of labelling and packaging

The label is an important element in the quality assurance of medicines. The label must be affixed to all over-the-counter medicines. However, all pharmaceutical preparations must comply with the labelling standards specified in good manufacturing practice. The following information must appear on the container label:

► Drug name ;

► Active substance content ;

► List of excipients ;

► Method of use and route(s) of administration ;

► Special warning that the medicine must be kept out of the sight and reach of children;

► Expiry date ;

► Special storage precautions ;

► Marketing authorisation number ;

► Batch number ;

► Instructions for use ;

► Name and address of manufacturer (27).

8.2. Thin film chromatography

This is a planar chromatography method in which the mobile phase is a liquid. It is used to separate or purify compounds. It works simply. A plate is a glass or aluminium support coated on one side with a stationary phase in a uniform layer. This stationary phase is usually silica. It is possible to add a fluorescence agent to allow ultraviolet reading if the compounds in the sample are not coloured. At the start of the analysis, a pencil line is drawn horizontally one centimetre from the bottom of the TLC plate. Then, using a capillary, deposits are made on the line drawn. These deposits correspond to the sample to be analysed and the comparison controls. At the same time, the eluent or mobile phase is prepared in a 5 mm high glass vat and the vat is left to reach saturation. The plate is then placed upright (vertically) in the tank and the compounds are carried away by capillary action, following the migration of the eluent on the plate. When the eluent reaches the top of the plate, the plate is removed from the tank and the solvent front is marked with a line. The eluent is left to evaporate. The migrations are then revealed. This can be done under ultraviolet light if the mobile phase contains a fluorescent agent, by spraying the plate with vanillin or by spraying with potassium permanganate. By comparison with the controls (if the migration of a compound is at the same level as that of a control) we can then conclude as to the identity of the different components or we can highlight impurities.

o **Front-end ratio and advantages of CCM**

The front ratio (R_f) expresses the ratio between the distance covered by the substance and the distance covered by the mobile phase front.

distance travelled by the substance

$$R_f = \frac{distance\ parcourue\ par\ la\ substance}{distance\ parcourue\ par\ le\ front\ du\ solvant}$$

These distances are measured from the starting line corresponding to the centre of the initial deposit of the mixture to be separated to the centre of the spot(s) and the solvent front. It should be noted that each substance has an R_f in a given chromatographic system.

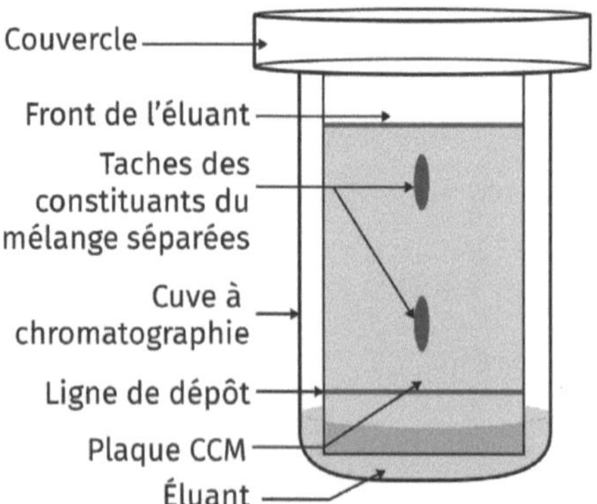

Figure 3: Diagram illustrating how CCM works

8.3. Analysis techniques for determining the content of product components

Analytical chemistry is a branch of chemistry that enables "the constituents of a sample of matter to be separated, identified and their respective quantities determined. Qualitative analysis reveals the chemical nature of the substances present. Quantitative analysis makes it possible to quantify the relative importance of one or more of them, called analytes".

8.3.1. tirage dosing

Dosing (or titrating) a chemical species (molecule or ion) in solution means determining its molar concentration in the solution in question. In the case of a destructive or direct assay, a chemical reaction is used. A titrating solution containing a titrant chosen according to the species to be determined is used. The solutions are placed as shown in the diagram opposite:

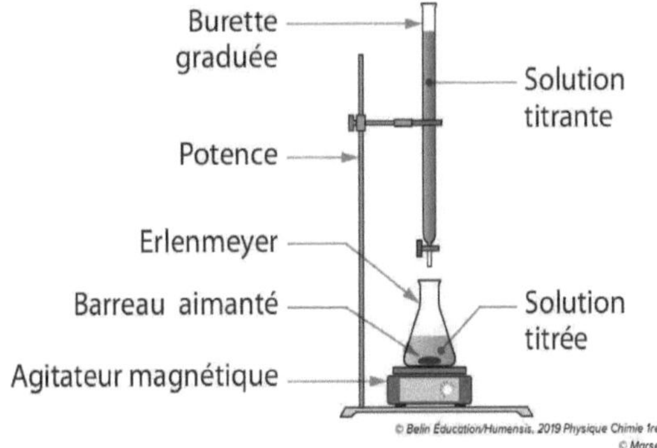

Figure 4: Chemical titration diagram

8.3.2. UV-Visible spectrometry :

The ultraviolet-visible spectrometer (UV-Vis) is defined as an optical system capable of producing monochromatic radiation in the range 200 to 780 nm and as a device capable of detecting optical transmission, usually expressed as absorbance (A), whose main function is to measure the absorbance or transmission declared at one or more defined wavelengths.

A UV-Vis spectrometer may also be called a spectrophotometer or absorption spectrometer (28).

✦ **Principle**

UV-Visible spectroscopy is performed using a spectrophotometer. When the cell containing the solution is placed in a spectroscope, it receives radiation of intensity I0; some of this incident light, I_0 , is absorbed by the medium and the rest, I, is transmitted. The intensity (I) of the radiation from the cuvette is therefore less than the intensity of the initial radiation (I_0). The fraction of incident light absorbed by a substance of concentration C contained in a cell of length l is given by Beer-Lambert's law:

$DO = A = \log(I_0 /I) = s \, l \, C$

s: molar extinction coefficient.

A: specific absorbance of a dissolved substance, refers to the absorbance of a 10 g/L solution at a thickness of 1 cm at a given wavelength (28).

In Beer-Lambert's law, the absorbance (A) or optical density (OD) of a solution at a given wavelength, $\grave{A}$, is defined as the logarithm to the base 10 of the inverse of the transmittance (T) for monochromatic radiation.

It is expressed by the following equation:

$$A = \log 10 \; x\frac{1}{T} = \log 10 \frac{I_0}{I} \; \textbf{avec} \; T = \frac{I}{I_0}$$

Io: Intensity of incident monochromatic radiation; I: Intensity of transmitted monochromatic radiation.

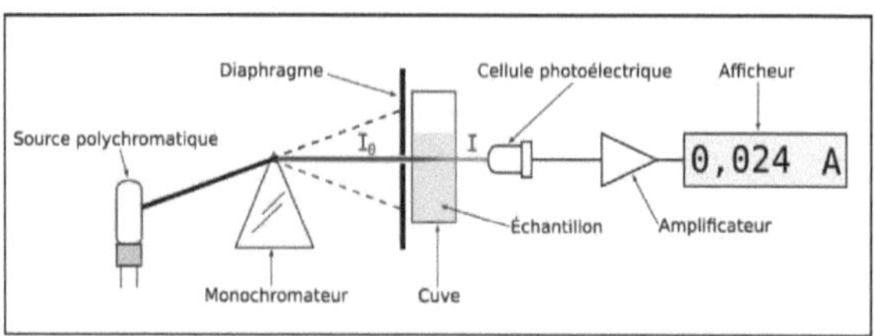

Figure 5: Schematic diagram of the UV-visible single-beam spectrophotometer.

8.3.3. High performance liquid chromatography (HPLC) :

HPLC is a method for separating the constituents of a mixture, which may be simple or complex. It is used to identify and quantify the constituents of a mixture (29). HPLC is described in the diagram below.

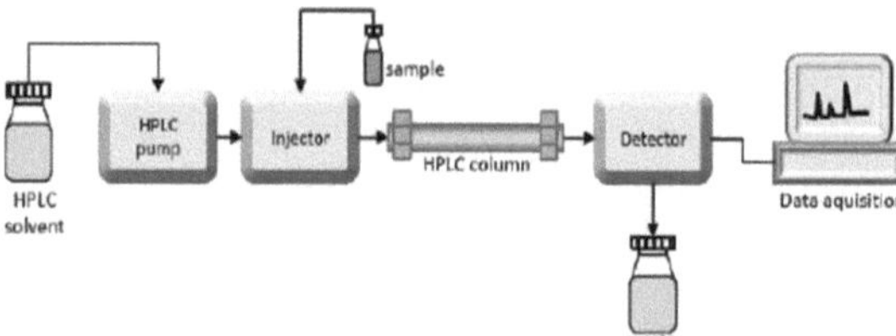

Figure 6: Diagram showing how HPLC works

The sample to be injected must be prepared in such a way that the liquid phase is clear and free from of particles. Micro-extraction can be carried out during preparation.A tank of liquid mobile phase is connected to a pump. This mobile phase is used as the eluent, which draws the sample into the system. Several bottles of eluent (solvents of different polarities) can be used to create elution gradients, i.e. gradually changing the polarity of the mobile phase using the pump. The pump is used to control the flow rate of the mobile phase, as well as programming the elution gradients of the different solvents connected to it. You can work in isocratic mode (with 100% of the same solvent) or in gradient mode (with a variation in the concentration of the mixture of eluents).

The sample is injected via an injection valve consisting of an injection loop of known volume. This system ensures a constant injection volume, which is important for quantitative analysis. Injections can be carried out manually, but automatic samplers are now widely used in laboratories to save time. The sample is then carried by the mobile phase through the column, which is made of inert material (stainless steel or glass). The internal diameter is constant (4 to 20 mm) and the length is generally between 15 and 30 cm. The column contains a stationary phase that allows compounds to be separated by retention. Two types of phase are possible:

o **The normal phase** consists of silica gel, which is a very polar material. To avoid interactions between the mobile phase and the stationary phase, an apolar mobile phase must be used. In this way, the polar compounds in the sample will be retained more than the non-polar compounds, which will then come out of the column first. However, the mobile phase must have a certain polarity to prevent polar compounds from being retained too much in the column.

o **The reverse phase**, which contains silica grafted with carbon chains generally containing 8 or 18 carbon atoms. This phase is therefore apolar and the use of a polar mobile phase is necessary. Here it is the polar compounds that are eluted first. The polarity of the mobile phase must also be adjusted to prevent apolar compounds from being retained too much.

METHODOLOGY

1. Framework

1.1. Framework

The study is taking place at the National Health Laboratory (LNS), a public scientific and technological establishment. According to article 2 of order N°00-40/P- RM of 20 September 2000 creating the LNS, it is responsible for controlling the quality of medicines, foods and beverages and other substances produced or imported into the Republic of Mali and intended for therapeutic, dietetic or dietary purposes with a view to safeguarding the health of human and animal populations.

The LNS is made up of three main technical departments:

√ Drug Quality Control Department ;

√ Food and drink quality control department ;

√ Water quality control department.

The study will be carried out in the drug quality control department, which has all the equipment needed for drug analysis.

1.2. Type of study

This is a descriptive, analytical, cross-sectional study of the quality of injectable gentamicin dispensed in health centres and private pharmacies in Bamako.

1.3. Period of study

Our study took place over a period extending from 25 November 2022 to 30 September 2023 in the drug quality control department (SCQM) of the Laboratoire National de la Santé (LNS).

1.4. Population study

1.4.1. Inclusion criteria

The study concerns only gentamicin injection samples analysed during the study period.

1.4.2. Non-inclusion criteria

Samples analysed before and after the study period and out-of-date batches will not be included.

1.4.3. Sampling method

Our study focused on gentamycin sold in health centres and certain pharmacies in BAMAKO. The total number of samples to be taken was calculated using the MedRS (30). This tool calculates the number of samples with a confidence interval of 95%. On the basis of these analyses, 53 samples were collected, as shown in the attached table. All samples taken were labelled and coded in accordance with the LNS sampling plan. A sample collection form was completed for each sample, including the following information:

► The sampling date ;

► Sampling location ;

► The quantity taken ;

► Product designation ;

► Galenic form ;

► The batch number ;

► Dosage of active ingredient ;

► Date of manufacture ;

► Expiry date ;

► The manufacturing laboratory ;

► Regulatory status ;

► And the product's country of origin;

► Storage/climatic conditions at the sampling site/point (temperature and humidity, indication of daytime conditions only is acceptable, comments on suitability of premises where products are stored at the particular site. The samples taken were packaged, transported and stored in such a way as to avoid any deterioration, breakage or contamination and transported in their original container and in accordance with the storage instructions for the product concerned, from the collection site to the LNS. These samples were stored in the LNS sample library at a temperature < 25°C, protected from light, and then tested within the expiry date in accordance with Good Storage Practice. The difficulties and limitations of our study include the reluctance of some health workers to take samples, the administrative burden of obtaining approval prior to sampling, and the size of the sample.

1.4.4. Collection techniques and tools

Sampling was carried out using probability sampling based on reliable estimates and statistically valid calculations according to the LNS sampling plan.

1.5. Tools for processing and entering data

Data was entered using Word and Excel and processed using SPSS version 20 software.

1.6. Ethical considerations

The study was conducted in accordance with the principles of Good Laboratory Practice in force, the general requirements concerning the competence of calibration and testing laboratories (ISO 17025) and the strict confidentiality of the results of the analysis.

1.7. Quality control methods for gentamicin injectable

The assessment was carried out in accordance with British Pharmacopoeia (BP) standards using test methods (pH, Mean Volume), identification methods (Thin Layer Chromatography, Minilab®) and assays (UV-Visible Spectrophotometry). In addition to these British Pharmacopoeia methods, other methods were used (Manufacturer's Dossier, In-house Methods).

1.7.1. Tests

► **Visual examination**

The primary and secondary packaging of the various brands was carefully examined to verify the required information, such as the product name, manufacturer's address, date of manufacture, batch number, expiry date, active ingredient content and registration number.

► **Determination of Average Volume :**

⤶ **Interest**

The US Pharmacopoeia specifies that the average volume is used to provide assurance that oral liquids, when transferred from the original container, will provide the volume of dosage form declared on the label. The average volume of liquid obtained from the 10 containers is not less than 100% and the volume of any container is less than 95% of the volume declared in the labelling (31).

⤶ **Principle**

This involves emptying the ampoule as completely as possible and determining the mass or volume of its contents, as appropriate. In the case of emulsions and suspensions, shake the container before determination. The result obtained must not be less than the value indicated on the label.(32)

► **Determination of pH** ⤶ **Why :**

It is often observed that the tolerance, stability and efficacy of a product vary with the pH. It is therefore important to choose a pH that is not too poorly tolerated, while still ensuring acceptable stability of the active ingredient.

⤶ **Principle :**

The pH meter was calibrated with buffer solutions of pH 2.0, 4.0 and 7.0. The contents of 5 ampoules were emptied into a beaker. The pH was measured by inserting the pH meter electrode into the drug solution and the reading was taken after stabilisation. This was done in duplicate and the procedure repeated for each sample.

The pH of gentamycin injection is between 3.0 and 5.5 according to the British Pharmacopoeia (33).

► **Identification method**

To identify the active ingredient, we used the Minilab® technique from GPHF. The spot obtained from the test solution must correspond in terms of colour, size, intensity, shape and displacement distance (relative retention factor) to that of the chromatogram obtained with the standard solution and with no additional spots indicating the presence of undeclared compounds or contaminants according to the formula: (31).

$$\%Rf = \frac{RfStd - RfEch}{RfStd} * 100 \leq 5\%$$

1.7.2. Dosage :

► **UV-visible spectroscopy (AGILENT 8453) :**

Absorbances were read using an Agilent 8453 spectrophotometer equipped with a 1024-element PDA (Agilent Technologies, Germany). All spectra were recorded using the UV-Vis wavelength range from 200 to 500 nm. The acquired data was processed using Chemstation software.

Procedure :

For all standard solutions and samples, a 0.1N NaOH solution was used as the solvent.
Since the optical density was found to be highest in the spectrum at 217 nm, quantification was carried out at this wavelength.

• **Preparation of the standard**: the reference substance was gentamicin sulphate as a pure powder from the British Pharmacopoeia.

A sheet of aluminium foil was placed on the measuring pan of the electronic pocket balance; after being set to zero, exactly 0.0144g approximately of the reference substance corresponding to 10mg gentamycin sulphate was measured using a spatula. Carefully empty the aluminium foil into a 10mL volumetric flask and drain off all the solid residue with 10mL of 0.1N NaOH using a graduated pipette.

Seal the vial and place in an ultrasonic shaker until all the solids have dissolved. The final solution obtained should contain 1mg/ml gentamycin sulphate.

• **Sample preparation:** the sample was prepared under the same conditions as the standard with a final concentration of 1mg/mL gentamycin sulphate and 1N NaOH as solvent.

• **Method validation:** Before a method is used, it is essential that it be validated analytically to ensure that it is fit for purpose. We therefore undertook the analytical validation of the method in order to determine its precision, reproducibility and linearity. The initial results obtained allow the method to be used in the routine quality control of gentamycin injection at the LNS.

1.8. Interpretation

Results are considered non-compliant when all the determinations in the analytical protocol do not comply with the standards given in the following pharmacopoeias: British Pharmacopoeia, American Pharmacopoeia and International Pharmacopoeia.

RESULTS

During this study, 20 cases of non-compliance were recorded out of the 53 samples analysed, representing a rate of 38%. The samples were classified according to several criteria:

o Sampling location ;

o Country of manufacture ;

o The name on the box ;

o Registration status ;

o The active ingredient ;

o Depending on the quality of the samples (Average volume, pH, UV/visible spectrophotometer, TLC).

Table II: Breakdown of samples by sampling sector

Sector	Workforce	Percentage (%)
PRIVATE DISPENSARY	32	60,4
CSCOM	11	20,7
HOSPITAL	4	7,5
CSREF	3	5,7
LNS	3	5,7
Total	53	100

The private sector is the one with the highest deduction rate, at 60.4%.

Table III: Breakdown of samples by country of origin

Provenance	Effectif	Pourcentage (%)
CHINE	35	66,0
TOGO	9	17,0
INDE	9	17,0
Total	53	100,0

China is the country with the largest sample of origins.

Table IV: Distribution of samples by name on the box

Sector		Workforce	Percentage (%)
	Gentamycin	40	75,4
	Gentamycin TM	9	17,0
	Gentamycin sixer	2	3,8
	Genglob	1	1,9
	Devgentam	1	1,9
	Total	53	100

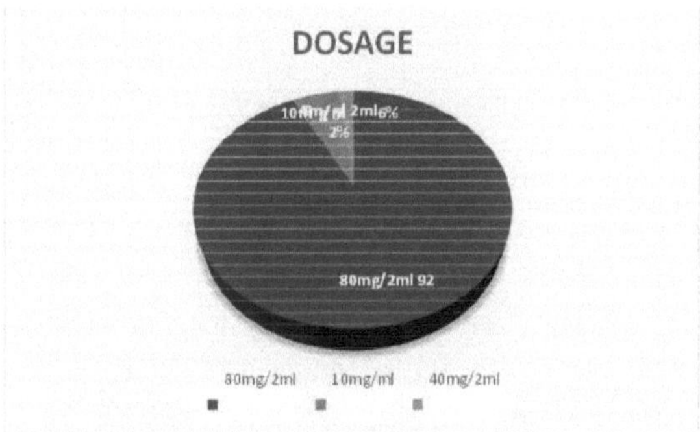

Figure 7: Distribution of samples by assay.

Gentamicin sulphate 80mg/2ml is the most widely represented with a rate of 92%.

Table V: Breakdown of samples by registration status

DESIGNATION	Workforce	Percentage (%)
Invalid MA	42	79,0
Valid MA	11	21,0
Total	53	100

Over 79% of samples had invalid marketing authorisations.

Table VI: Distribution of samples according to average volume compliance

VM compliance	Workforce	Percentage (%)
Compliant	51	96,2
Non-compliant	2	3,8
Total	53	100

The non-compliance rate is 3.8% according to average volume compliance

Table VII: Distribution of samples according to pH compliance

pH compliance	Workforce	Percentage (%)
Compliant	48	90,6
Non-compliant	5	9,4
Total	53	100

The rate of non-compliance was 9.4% for pH compliance

Table VIII: Distribution of samples according to TLC compliance

CCM compliance	Workforce	Percentage (%)
Compliant	53	100,0
Non-compliant	0	0
Total	53	100

All samples conform to TLC

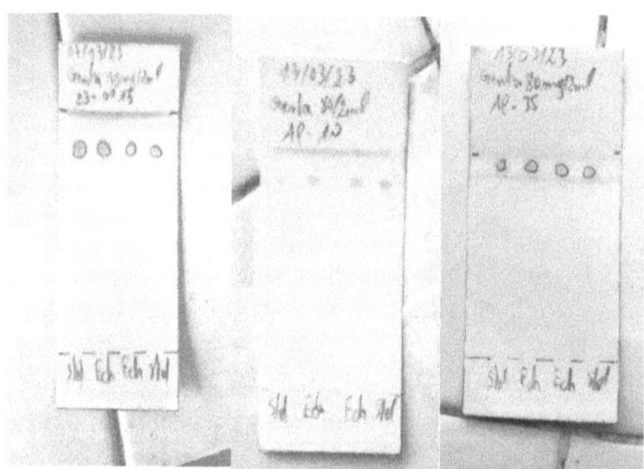

Figure 8: some compliant TLC plates

Table IX: Distribution of samples according to compliance by UV/visible spectroscopy

Spectro UV compliance	Workforce	Percentage (%)
Compliant	36	67,9
Non-compliant	17	32,1
Total	53	100

The non-compliance rate was 32.1% for UV/visible spectroscopy.

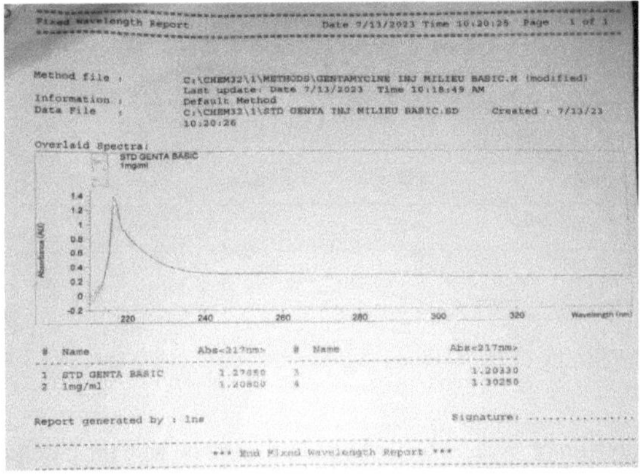

Figure 9: Assay spectrum of the standard

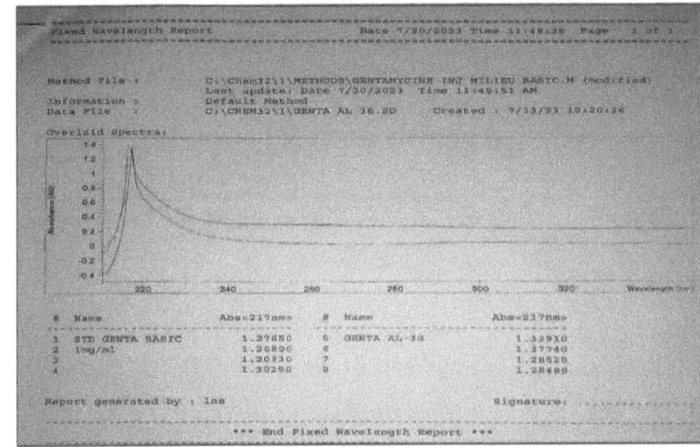

Figure 10: Assay spectrum of sample AL-36

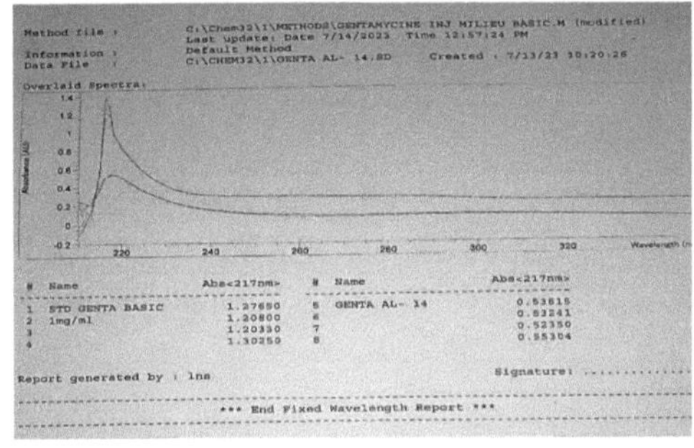

Figure 11: Assay spectrum of sample AL-14

Table X: Distribution of samples according to the compliance of the Uv-visible spectro in relation to the average volume

Visible uv spectro **Total**

	Compliant	Non-compliant	
Compliant	34	17	51
Non-compliant	2	0	2
Total	36	17	53

Samples not conforming to the average volume are conforming to the Uv-visible spectro.

Table XI: Distribution of samples according to compliance with the Uv-visible spectro in relation to pH

Visible uv spectro **Total**

	Compliant	Non-compliant	
Compliant	35	13	48
Non-compliant	1	4	5
Total	36	17	53

4 samples that did not comply with the pH test did not comply with the Uv-visible spectro test.

Table XII: Distribution of samples according to compliance with average volume in relation to pH

	VM		Total
	Compliant	Non-compliant	
Compliant	46	2	48
Non-compliant	5	0	5
Total	51	2	53

Samples that do not comply with the pH are compliant with the average volume.

Table XIII: Overall non-compliance situation

Overall compliance	Workforce	Percentage (%)
Compliant	33	62,0
Non-compliant	20	38,0
Total	53	100

Overall, 20 samples were non-compliant, i.e. 38%.

Table XIV: Distribution of samples according to conformity by country of origin

Country		Global		Total
	Non-compliant		Compliant	
China	14		21	35
India	5		4	9
Togo	1		8	9
Total	20		33	53

China is the country with the highest rate of non-conforming samples.
68.42% of the total

Table XV: Breakdown of samples by registration and compliance status

AMM		Global		Total
	Non-compliant		Compliant	
Invalid	19		23	42
Valid	1		10	11
Total	20		33	53

Overall, 19 non-compliant samples (95%) had invalid MA.

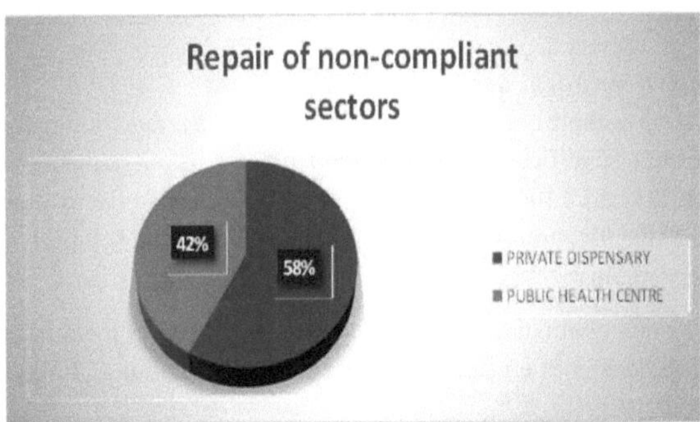

Figure 12: Breakdown of non-compliant samples by sampling sector

COMMENTS AND DISCUSSION

1. Limits of the study

Our study covered all samples taken in health facilities and private dispensaries in Bamako during the study period, in accordance with the LNS programme of activities. Like all human work, ours was confronted with shortcomings:

- Unavailability of the product in certain health centres;

- The categorical refusal of certain structures to take part in the study;

- Not all reagents were available to perform the HPLC method.

2. Summary of analytical methods

The various analysis methods used for this study included: Method

and pharmaceutical quality.

2.1. Physical and chemical analysis

All samples complied with good manufacturing practice when the packaging and labels of the primary and secondary packaging of the various samples used for analysis were inspected in accordance with USP specifications.

The results obtained for physico-chemical analysis, pH and TLC were analysed against USP and BP specifications. The pH of the product may reflect the intrinsic pH of the active pharmaceutical ingredient. In this study, out of 53 samples, 5 were not pH compliant. All samples were TLC compliant.

2.2. Analysis of pharmaceutical quality⁺ Average volume

In our study, out of 53 samples, 2 did not comply with the average volume according to the British Pharmacopoeia specifications for volume uniformity of single-dose preparations, which are between 90 and 110%. The causes of non-conformity were due to the average volume being out of specification (higher or lower than the average volume).

⁺ UV-Visible spectroscopy

This is a quantitative and qualitative analytical method that involves measuring the absorbance or optical density of a given chemical substance in solution. It requires great care in dilution and pipetting.

The method presented is based on the ability of gentamicin to form complex combinations that absorb UV-Visible light in 1N NaOH medium and at a final concentration of 1 mg/mL of the sample after dilution. It obeys Lambert Beer's law and can therefore be used to determine gentamicin sulphate. Determination of the active ingredient content showed that 36 samples complied with the specifications required by the British Pharmacopoeia standard, with a range of drug content from 90% to 110%. The causes of non-compliance were due to under-dosage as well as over-dosage of active ingredient.

2.3. Quality of data

Non-compliant samples were subject to OOS treatment in accordance with the laboratory's procedure describing the management of out-of-specification results. All data was submitted

42

for review and approval by the laboratory's quality control functions in accordance with our technical file control procedure, which describes the specific provisions of the certificate of analysis and control required before final approval.

3. Summary of results

A total of 53 samples were taken or received and analysed according to a risk-based protocol, of which 33 were compliant and 20 non-compliant. These samples contained gentamicin sulphate in doses of 80 mg/2mL, 10 mg/mL and 40 mg/2mL and came mainly from the private sector (60.4%), followed by the public sector (39.6%). These results differ from those of Dembélé et al. who found 70% for the public sector and 30% for the private sector in a study on pharmaceutical quality assurance of injectable diazepam (34). This difference can be explained by the methodology used.

China was the largest country of origin of samples with a rate of 66%, followed by Togo and India with 17% each. These results differ from those of **Romain SIKA** in his study: Evaluation de la qualité du diazépam injectable prélevé dans les centres de santé et officines privées au mali en 2022, which found that India accounted for 65.1%, followed by France 21.1% and China 13.8% (35). These results differ from those of the PMS in recent years (36-38). This difference could be explained by the difference in methodology.

This study revealed that 79% of the samples had invalid MAs. This result confirms that of Dembele et al. who also found in a study on the pharmaceutical quality assurance of Diazepam injection that all the samples of Diazepam injection were not registered or had an invalid MA (34). This could explain the high rate of non-compliance obtained in our study (38%) and that of Dembele et al. This result is also close to that of the Working Group on Child Health, which found a non-compliance rate of 41% in an international study on the quality of injectable gentamicin (39). This result could be explained by non-compliance with the Schéma Directeur d'Approvisionnement et de Distribution des Médicaments Essentiels et autres Produits de Santé (SDADME-PS).In our study, the private sector accounted for 58% of non-compliant samples and the public sector for 42%. These results differ from those of Romain SIKA and SIDIBE, who found that 20% and 80% came from the private and public sectors respectively (13,35). The causes of non-compliance were due to an underdose of active ingredient, an overdose of active ingredient and/or an average volume or pH out of specification.Of the non-compliant samples, 14 came from China, 5 from India and 1 from Togo, equivalent in percentage terms to 70%, 25% and 5% respectively. In addition, the majority of samples with a pH out of specification were non-compliant by UV-visible spectroscopy. The UV-visible spectroscopy revealed that some samples that conformed according to TLC were non-conforming. This can be explained by the fact that TLC is an identification method that can detect even traces of the active ingredient, unlike UV-visible spectroscopy, which is a method for quantifying the active ingredient.

CONCLUSION AND RECOMMENDATIONS

1. CONCLUSION

Guaranteeing the quality of pharmaceutical products, whether manufactured locally or imported, is fundamental to any healthcare system. The use of ineffective, poor-quality and harmful medicines can lead to therapeutic failure, disease exacerbation, drug resistance and even death. It also contributes to reducing consumer confidence in healthcare systems, healthcare providers, manufacturers and distributors of pharmaceutical products.

At the end of our study on the evaluation of the quality of injectable gentamicin dispensed in health centres and private pharmacies in Bamako, we found that non-compliance affected both the private and public sectors. All the samples taken were unregistered or had their marketing authorisation expired, and came mainly from China and India.

The causes of non-compliance were due to either an underdose of active ingredient, an overdose of active ingredient and/or an average volume or pH out of specification.

The results clearly raise the issue of the systematic registration of medicines before they are placed on the market, compliance with the Master Plan for the Supply and Distribution of Essential Medicines and other Health Products, and the importance of ongoing quality control and post-marketing surveillance of medicines.

2. RECOMMENDATIONS

At the end of this work we make the following recommendations:

► AT THE NATIONAL HEALTH LABORATORY (LNS)

• Extend this study to the whole country for a large number of samples.

• Systematically send non-compliant analysis results to the DPM for action to be taken.

• Strengthen the capacity of the LNS.

► PHARMACY AND MEDICINES DEPARTMENT

• Ensuring compliance with the Essential Drug Supply Master Plan

and other Health Products (SDADME-PS).

• Set up an effective early warning coordination mechanism between the various

actors.

• Strengthen post-marketing control of medicines and other health products.

• Regularly update the marketing authorisation data for medicinal products.

► THE HEALTH INSPECTORATE

• Ensuring compliance with Good Storage Practices for pharmaceutical products throughout the distribution chain.

BIBLIOGRAPHY

1. Diop A, Sarr SO, Diop YM, Niang AA, Ndiaye B. [Control of the quality of cotrimoxazole medicines used in Senegal]. Therapie. 1 Sept 2008;63(5):405-8.
2. Study of the socio-economic and public health impact of low-quality medical products inferior and falsified medical products [Internet]. [cited 25 Sept 2023]. Available from on: https://www.who.int/fr/publications-detail/a-study-on-the-public-health-and- socioeconomic-impact-of-substandard-and-falsified-medical-products
3. Access to medicines and vaccines.

4. Establishment of the African Medicines Agency: progress, challenges and regulatory readiness - PubMed [Internet]. [cited 25 Sep 2023]. Available from: https://pubmed.ncbi.nlm.nih.gov/33685518/
5. Appel GB, Neu HC. Gentamicin in 1978. Ann Intern Med. 1978;89(4):528-38.

6. Gres E. Antibiotic prescribing practices according to the AWARE classification in children under five years of age at decentralised and hospital level in West Africa (2021-2022).
7. mali_nap_2019_2023.pdf [Internet]. [cited 12 Jan. 2024]. Available at: https://cdn.who.int/media/docs/default-source/antimicrobial-resistance/amr-spc-npm/nap-library/mali_nap_2019_2023.pdf?sfvrsn=a767a737_1&download=true
8. Draft_01_final_Manuel_SDADME_PS_2021 (3).docx.

9. Begert L. Drug packaging: an essential element of patient protection. :127.
10. What are the different names of medicines? [Internet]. [cited 29 Oct 2022]. Available from: https://www.weka.fr/sante/dossier-pratique/maitrise-des-risques-et-de-la- qualite-dt86/quelles-sont-les-differentes-denominations-des-medicaments-5225/
11. The different names for medicines and which one to use? - Réussis ton IFSI [Internet]. [cited 25 Sep 2023]. Available from: https://reussistonifsi.fr/denominations- medicaments/

12. Galenic pharmacy _ Good manufacturing practice for medicinal products (PDFDrive.com).pdf.

13. SIDIBE OI. Quality control of antimalarial drugs in 7 regions administratives du Mali. 2011;1-99.

14. MEDBOX | Counterfeit Medicines - Guide to the development of measures to combat... [Internet]. [cited 17 Jan 2024]. Available on:

https://www.medbox.org/document/medicaments-contrefaits-guide-pour-lelaboration-de-mesures-visant-a-eliminer-les-medicaments-contrefaits#GO
15. Substandard and falsified medical products [Internet]. [cited 27 Oct 2023]. Available from: https://www.who.int/news-room/fact-sheets/detail/substandard-and-falsified-medical- products
16. What is a generic drug? - ANSM : Agence nationale de sécurité du médicament et des produits de santé [Internet]. [cited 15 Jan 2024]. Available from: https://archive.ansm.sante.fr/Dossiers/Medicaments-generiques/Qu-est-ce-qu-un- medicament-generique/(offset)/0
17. Bryskier A. Antibiotics, antibacterial and antifungal agents. ELLIPSES; 1999.

18. Byrn S, Clase K, Ekeocha Z, Masekela F. Product Information Report. 2022;(March).

19. Plus M. Gentamicin Injection Job Aid to Assist with Laboratory Testing. 2023;(April).

20. Budd E, Cramp E, Sharland M, Hand K, Howard P, Wilson P, et al. Adaptation of the WHO Essential Medicines List for national antibiotic stewardship policy in England: being AWaRe. J Antimicrob Chemother. 1 Nov 2019;74(11):3384-9.

21. Emmanuel AS, Qualite CDE, Medicaments DES, Toliara DLE province DE. ANDRIANANTENAINTSOLO Samuel Emmanuel CONTROLE DE QUALITE DES MEDICAMENTS ANTIPALUDIQUES DANS L'EX-PROVINCE DE TOLIARA Thesis Doctorate in Medicine.

22. Truchaud A, Cazaubiel M, Dik M, Le Neel T, and Lustenberge... - Google Scholar [Internet]. [cited 30 Oct 2022]. Available at: https://scholar.google.com/scholar?hl=fr&as_sdt=0%2C5&q=Truchaud+A%2C+Cazaubi el+M%2C+Dik+M%2C+Le+Neel+T%2C+and+Lustenberger+P.+L%27assurance+quality+. %3A&btnG=

23. TRS 986 - Annex 3: WHO model quality assurance system for procurement agencies [Internet]. [cited 19 Oct 2023]. Available from: https://www.who.int/fr/publications/m/item/trs-986-annex-3

24. WHO Good Manufacturing Practice for Pharmaceuticals: Main Principles [Internet]. [cited 19 Oct 2023]. Available from at: https://www.who.int/publications/m/item/bonnes-pratiques-de-fabrication-pour-les- substances-actives-pharmaceutiques

25. for WEC on S. WHO Expert Committee on Specifications for Preparations pharmaceuticals: twenty-seventh. 1980;

26. WHO G. Quality assurance of pharmaceutical products. Compendium of guidelines and other documents. v.1. 1998;

27. Tièmoko MD. Quality control of antiretroviral drugs at the National Health Laboratory of Mali. Univ Sci Tech Technol Bamako. 2011;88.

28. USP-NF {857) Ultraviolet-Visible Spectroscopy [Internet]. [cited 16 March 2023]. Available from: https://online.uspnf.com/uspnf/document/1_GUID-4C5C1937-524A-4BED-95E7-384EDE3745E0_4_en-US?source=TOC

29. Ranger J. Analytical Control techniques adapted to the fight against counterfeit medicines. 2015;109.

30. MEDRSPROD | Sample Size Calculator [Internet]. [cited 25 Oct 2023]. Available from: https://pqmplustools.com/medrsprod/Home/VIEwoNLY/samplesizecalculator/lookup

31. Evaluation of the quality of injectable diazepam drawn from health centres and private pharmacies in Mali 2022-2023.

32. Study of non-compliant medicines at the national health laboratory from 1 January to 31 December 2016.

33. Medsafe. Gentamicin Injection Datasheet. 2019;(2):42020.

34. Pharmaceutical Quality Assurance of Diazepam Injection at the National Health Laboratory of Mali | International Journal of Pharmaceutical and Bio Medical Science. 24 Dec 2022 [cited 18 Jan 2023]; Available from:

https://ijpbms.com/index.php/ijpbms/article/view/215

35. Sika KTJR. Evaluation of the quality of injectable diazepam taken from health centres and private pharmacies in Mali in 2022. [Internet] [Thesis]. USTTB; 2023 [cited 15 Jan 2024]. Available from: https://www.bibliosante.ml/handle/123456789/12171

36. Dembélé O, Coulibaly S, Dakouo J, Koumaré B. PRE- AND POST-MARKETING CONTROL OF DRUG QUALITY AT THE NATIONAL HEALTH LABORATORY, BAMAKO-MALI. Univers J Pharm Res. 15 Jan 2022;

37. Dembele O, Coulibaly SM, Cissé BM, Cissé M, Dakouo J, Cissé NH, et al. Risk-Based Post-Marketing Surveillance (RB-PMS) of antimalarial drugs and maternal, neonatal and reproductive health (MNCH) in Mali. J Drug Deliv Ther. 7 March 2022;12(2):6-10.

38. Risk-Based Post-Marketing Surveillance (RB-PMS2) of Antimalarial and MNCH drugs in Mali (PY2) | International Journal of Pharmaceutical and Bio Medical Science. 27 Sep 2022 [cited 30 Mar 2023]; Available from: https://ijpbms.com/index.php/ijpbms/article/view/146

39. Health C, Force T. medicines for newborn and child health for primary health care : pediatric amoxicillin and gentamicin. 2022;

Appendix I: Example of a data collection form

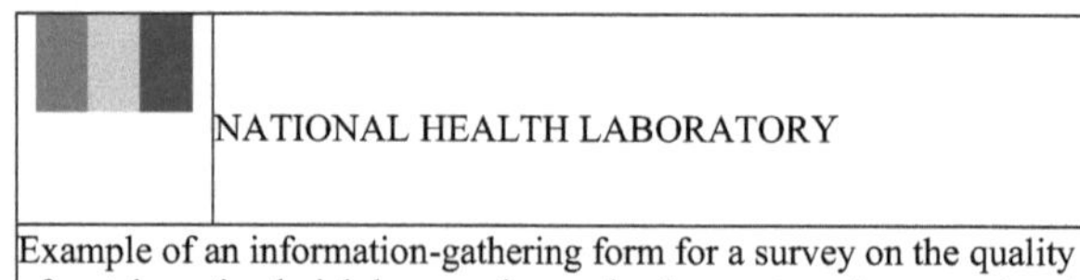

<table>
<tr><td></td><td>NATIONAL HEALTH LABORATORY</td></tr>
<tr><td colspan="2">Example of an information-gathering form for a survey on the quality of certain antimalarial drugs and reproductive, maternal, neonatal and infant health drugs in circulation in Mali</td></tr>
</table>

Unique sample code : (Name of region/facility identification number) (A: B)
Type of collection point: Private :; Public: ; NGO: Name of the point of sale of the medicine/place where the sample was taken:
Address (including telephone number, fax number and e-mail address, if applicable):
Name of the sample product:
Name of active pharmaceutical ingredient(s) (INN) with strength:
Pharmaceutical form (tablet, capsule, powder for injection, etc.):
Packaging size, type and material of container:
Batch/lot number:
Date of manufacture:
Expiry date:
Regulatory status in the country, registration number, if applicable:
Name and address of manufacturer:
Quantity collected (number of sample units or multi-dose containers taken) :
Storage/climatic conditions at sampling site/point (temperature and humidity, indication of daytime conditions only is acceptable, comments on suitability of premises where products are stored on the site particular for information at the DPM
Any anomalies, remarks or observations that may be considered relevant:

Date sample taken :
Name and signature of samplers:
Name and signature of Supervisor :
Please note:
✓ The samples taken must remain in their original containers, intact and unopened.
✓ This sample information collection form must always be kept with the sample taken.
✓ Appropriate sampling procedures must be followed.
✓ The Excel database must be filled in correctly.

Annex II :

No	Code of samples	Brand name	Manufacturer	Batch number	Country of origin	Status registration	Result
1	AL-01	Gentamicin	SINO PHARMACEUTICAL EQUIPMENT CO.LTD	200548	China	Invalid MA	Pass
2	AL-02	Gentamicin	SINO PHARMACEUTICAL EQUIPMENT CO.LTD	201148	China	Invalid MA	Pass
3	AL-03	Gentamicin	Tong Mei Laboratory	90522	Togo	Invalid MA	Pass
4	AL-04	Gentamicin	SINO PHARMA	201148	China	Invalid MA	Pass
5	AL-05	Gentamicin	Kwality Pharmaceuticals ltd	N-16147	India	Invalid MA	Non-compliant
6	AL-06	Gentamicin	NORTH CHINA Pharmaceutical	220340	China	Invalid MA	Pass
7	AL-07	Gentamicin	Tong Mei Laboratory	90522	Togo	Valid MA	Non-compliant
8	AL-08	Gentamicin	Tong Mei Laboratory	140720	Togo	Valid MA	Pass
9	AL-09	Gentamicin	NORTH CHINA Pharmaceutical	220340	China	Invalid MA	Pass
10	AL-10	Gentamicin	NORTH CHINA Pharmaceutical	220340	China	Invalid MA	Pass
11	AL-11	Gentamicin	Farmasino pharmaceutical	FS210 10 7	China	Invalid MA	Pass
12	AL-12	Gentamicin	NORTH CHINA Pharmaceutical	220340	China	Invalid MA	Pass
13	AL-13	Gentamicin	NORTH CHINA Pharmaceutical	220340	China	Invalid MA	Pass
14	AL-14	Gentamicin	Pharma international	P200905	China	Invalid MA	Non-compliant
15	AL-15	Gentamicin	Tong Mei Laboratory	90522	Togo	Valid MA	Pass
16	AL-16	Gentamicin	NORTH CHINA Pharmaceutical	220340	China	Invalid MA	Pass
17	AL-18	Gentamicin	Tong Mei Laboratory	90522	Togo	Valid MA	Pass
18	AL-19	Gentamicin	Pharma international LTD	P200905	China	Invalid MA	Non-compliant
19	AL-20	Gentamicin	Guizhou Tiandi pharmaceutical	211034	China	Invalid MA	Non-compliant

20	AL-21	Gentamicin	NASBIC CORPORATION GROUP CO,LTD	210213	China	Invalid MA	Non-compliant
21	AL-22	Gentamicin	Tong Mei Laboratory	90522	Togo	Valid MA	Pass
22	AL-23	Gentamicin	Humanwell pharma mali	201126	China	Invalid MA	Pass
23	AL-24	Gentamicin	Humanwell pharma mali	200697	China	Invalid MA	Non-compliant
24	AL-25	Gentamicin	SINO PHARMACEUTICAL EQUIPMENT CO.LTD	200548	China	Invalid MA	Non-compliant
25	AL-26	Gentamicin	Trading private limited	S210245	India	Valid MA	Pass
26	AL-27	Gentamicin	Tianjin king york group hubei	210528	China	Invalid MA	Non-compliant
27	AL-28	Gentamicin	Tianjin king york group hubei	210528	China	Invalid MA	Non-compliant
28	AL-29	Gentamicin	Farmasino pharmaceutical	FS21010 7	China	Invalid MA	Pass
29	AL-30	Gentamicin	Humanwell pharma mali	210447	China	Invalid MA	Non-compliant
30	AL-31	Gentamicin	Guizhou Tiandi pharmaceutical	211034	China	Invalid MA	Non-compliant
31	AL-32	Gentamicin	NORTH CHINA Pharmaceutical	220340	China	Invalid MA	Pass
32	AL-33	Gentamicin	NORTH CHINA Pharmaceutical	220340	China	Invalid MA	Pass
33	AL-17	Gentamicin	Trading private limited	S210245	India	Valid MA	Pass
34	AL-34	Gentamicin	Tong Mei Laboratory	90522	Togo	Valid MA	Pass
35	AL-35	Gentamicin	Farmasino pharmaceutical	FS21010 7	China	Invalid MA	Pass
36	AL-36	Gentamicin	BENLEX TRADING PVT LTD	220456	India	Invalid MA	Pass
37	AL-37	Gentamicin	NORTH CHINA Pharmaceutical	220340	China	Invalid MA	Pass
38	AL-38	Gentamicin	DEVLIFO CORPORATION	31D2 2001	India	Invalid MA	Non-compliant
39	AL-39	Gentamicin	Tianjin king york group hubei	210528	India	Invalid MA	Non-compliant
40	AL-40	Gentamicin	NORTH CHINA Pharmaceutical	2021030	China	Invalid MA	Pass

				3			
41	AL-41	Gentamicin	SHAN DONG YIKANG PHARMACEUTICAL	210107	china	Invalid MA	Pass
42	AL-42	Gentamicin	Farmasino pharmaceutical	FS21020 7	China	Invalid MA	Pass
43	AL-43	Gentamicin	Tong Mei Laboratory	90522	Togo	Valid MA	Pass
44	AL-44	Gentamicin	Tianjin king york group hubei	210528	China	Invalid MA	Non-compliant
45	AL-45	Gentamicin	SHAN DONG YIKANG PHARMACEUTICAL	20210303	China	Invalid MA	Pass
46	AL-46	Gentamicin	Farmasino pharmaceutical	FS21010 7	China	Invalid MA	Pass
47	AL-47	Gentamicin	Tianjin king york group hubei	210528	China	Invalid MA	Non-compliant
48	AL-48	Gentamicin	Tong Mei Laboratory	90522	Togo	Valid MA	Pass
49	AL-49	Gentamicin	CHINA NATIONAL PHARMACEUTICAL GROUP	201148	china	Invalid MA	Pass
50	AL-50	Gentamicin	Kwality Pharmaceuticals ltd	N-16147	India	Invalid MA	Non-compliant
51	23-0013	Gentamicin	ACCELIUS GLOBAL	EL2201	India	Invalid MA	Non-compliant
52	22-0354	Gentamicin	Kwality Pharmaceuticals ltd	N-19719	India	Invalid MA	Non-compliant
53	23-0255	Gentamicin	Humanwell pharma mali	1012207 02	China	Invalid MA	Non-compliant

NAME: DAKOUO

FIRST NAME: Mawé Albert

Title of thesis :

EVALUATION OF THE QUALITY OF INJECTABLE GENTAMICIN DISPENSED IN HEALTH CENTRES AND PRIVATE PHARMACIES IN BAMAKO.

City where thesis was defended: Bamako

Depository: Faculty of Pharmacy Library.

Tel: 00223 73334495

E-MAIL: mawealbertdakouo@gmail.com

Sector of interest: quality control, pharmaceutical regulations, public health.

Summary of the thesis

Gentamicin is an aminoglycoside antibiotic produced by Micromonospora echinospora. It is a bactericidal inhibitor of protein synthesis. It is generally used as a curative treatment in combination with beta-lactam antibiotics. It may be prescribed as monotherapy in certain clinical situations, particularly in the treatment of Gram-negative bacterial infections. However, to guarantee therapeutic success, it is essential to use quality medicines in the current context of sub-standard, falsified and substandard medicines for essential multisource drugs.

The general aim of this study was to assess the quality of injectable gentamicin sold in health centres and private pharmacies in Bamako.

A total of 53 samples were taken, 32 from the private sector and 21 from the public sector (60.4% and 39.6% respectively). All the samples taken were unregistered or had expired marketing authorisations, and came mainly from China and India. After analysis, 20 samples did not comply with the required specifications. The causes of non-compliance were due to either an underdose of active ingredient, an overdose of active ingredient and/or an average volume or pH out of specification.

The results clearly raise the issue of the systematic registration of medicines before they are placed on the market, compliance with the Master Plan for the Supply and Distribution of Essential Medicines and other Health Products, and the importance of continuous quality control and post-marketing surveillance of medicines to ensure the health and guarantee access to quality medicines for the health and well-being of the population.

Key words: Quality control, Gentamicine, Bamako.

GALEN'S OATH

I swear, in the presence of the masters of the Faculty, the councillors of the Ordre des Pharmaciens, and of my fellow students: To honour those who have instructed me in the precepts of my art and to show them my gratitude. recognition by remaining faithful to their teaching;

To practise my profession conscientiously, in the interests of public health, and to comply not only with current legislation, but also with the rules of honour, probity and disinterestedness;

Never to forget my responsibility and my duties towards patients and their human dignity;

Under no circumstances will I agree to use my knowledge and status to corrupt the morals and encourage criminal acts;

May men esteem me if I am faithful to my promises. May I be covered and despised by my colleagues if I fail to do so!

I swear!

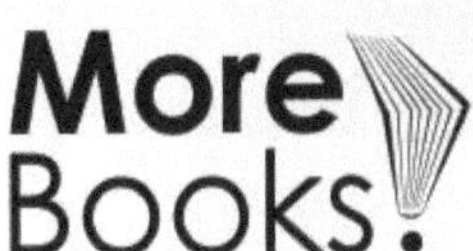

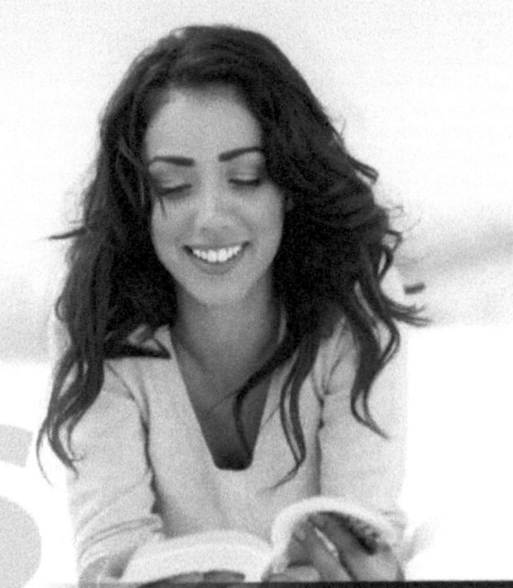

I want morebooks!

Buy your books fast and straightforward online - at one of world's fastest growing online book stores! Environmentally sound due to Print-on-Demand technologies.

Buy your books online at
www.morebooks.shop

Kaufen Sie Ihre Bücher schnell und unkompliziert online – auf einer der am schnellsten wachsenden Buchhandelsplattformen weltweit! Dank Print-On-Demand umwelt- und ressourcenschonend produziert.

Bücher schneller online kaufen
www.morebooks.shop

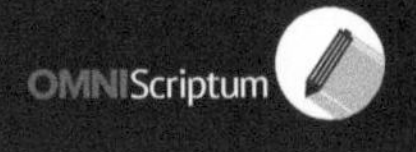

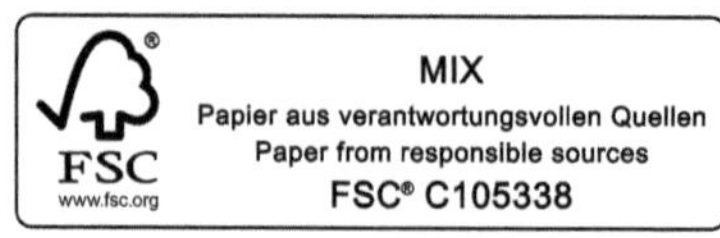

Printed by Books on Demand GmbH, Norderstedt / Germany